Losing with Evidence:
Your guide to developing an effective weight loss strategy

Losing with Evidence:
Your guide to developing an effective weight loss strategy

Micah Zuhl, Ph.D.

Micah Zuhl

2018

First Printing: 2018

ISBN 978-0-359-15057-1

Published by Micah Zuhl

mnzuhl@gmail.com

Ordering Information:

Special discounts are available on quantity purchases by corporations, associations, educators, and others. For details, contact the publisher at the above listed address.

Contents

Acknowledgements

To all of my colleagues, mentors, and teachers in the health and fitness field whose knowledge and guidance have supported my ability to develop this manual. To my fiancée, Taylor, for your continued and sustained support. You were the only one who routinely encouraged me to move forward with this project. Lastly, to my mother, who has been a pioneer in the health and fitness world as a teacher and practitioner. I am forever grateful to you for installing healthy behaviors into my early life.

Disclaimer

The information presented in this manual is intended for educational purposes only. You should not rely on this information as a substitute for professional medical advice, diagnosis, or treatment. You should consult your physician or other health care professional before starting this, or any other program.

Although the author has prepared this manual with diligence and accuracy to ensure completeness of information contained, he assumes no responsibility for errors, inaccuracies, omissions, or inconsistencies. Neither is any liability assumed for damages resulting from the use of the information contained herein.

Preface. How to use this manual

You may recall many years ago there existed a category of fictional books called "choose your own adventure". Nowadays, we have role playing video games in which the player decides their adventure within the story line of the game. This allows the player to make decisions about their character, and the enormous popularity of these types of games demonstrates that players want autonomy.

The intention of this manual is for you to choose your own weight loss strategy. Each of the strategies presented are evidence-based, which means they have been experimentally tested, and positive weight loss results have been demonstrated. Therefore, the strategies outlined in the manual are effective if incorporated into your life. For each one I will explain the concept, report results from several studies, and **present a template of how to follow the strategy**. In addition, I will provide pros and cons of the weight loss strategy.

I will also discuss the importance of exercise in combination with the weight loss and provide simple exercise recommendations. My hope is that you are able to develop a lifelong eating pattern that incorporates routine exercise, and that you ultimately achieve your weight loss goal.

Here is the challenge that I present to you...**READ THIS ENTIRE MANUAL**. It is not long and will take you approximately 30-40 minutes. Digest the information, and then develop your own weight loss strategy using the tools provided. This whole process will take 1-2 hours, and you will need a calculator. The framework is set, now dedicate yourself to improving your health.

About the author

I hold a doctorate degree in exercise physiology from the University of New Mexico (UNM). My research teams have conducted numerous studies on understanding the physiological responses to various types of exercise and nutritional supplements. I have also studied body composition techniques, along with exercise prescriptions for clinical populations (heart and neural disorders).

Additionally, in our research lab, we routinely measure resting metabolic rates among humans and use this information to assist them with achieving weight loss goals. We use science-based approaches to developing weight loss programs, which includes establishing calorie deficits in safe and practical ways.

I have also worked as both a clinical exercise physiologist and personal trainer. In these roles, I have prescribed exercise to improve cardiovascular and skeletal muscle function among both disease and healthy populations. I have also led educational seminars covering nutrition, dieting, exercise, and diseases.

I am also an educator and teach in various areas of exercise and health. A consistent topic of discussion with students is weight management, which typically turns into reviewing gimmick diets, which may be unsafe. This, combined with my previous experiences, has sparked my interest in developing a weight loss program that is easy to follow, effective, and grounded in research.

I hope you enjoy reading this manual, and able to utilize the information to develop your own weight loss strategy.

Your success is important to me, so please update me on your weight loss achievements @micahzuhl (Twitter), or zuhl09 (Instagram).

Section 1. Foundation dieting knowledge

Over the next several chapters I will introduce the concept of this manual and provide foundational knowledge on weight loss/gain and diet considerations. The goals of this section are to: (1) inform you about the physiological process of weight loss and gain; and (2) detail various dietary considerations such as a high protein approach. If you are uninterested and want to get right to the weight loss strategies then skip to section 2 of the manual

Chapter 1: Introduction

Let me start by saying that this manual is not a gimmick, scam, or some marketing ploy that I've developed to take your hard-earned money. I intend to provide you with a brief education on weight loss, and then present actual dietary strategies that have been studied by leading researchers in the field of weight loss. Throughout, I will refer to these as evidence-based weight loss strategies. These strategies do not require an investment in weekly meals, nutrient powders (e.g., shakes), or meetings. I will also not inundate you with my opinion, only with statistical supported results from studies using human participants. I will say that if you commit to one or several of these strategies then weight loss will be a likely outcome.

It has been estimated that 48% of women and 34% of men in the United States are trying to lose weight [1, 2]. I believe these percentages are much higher as many people (especially men) do not want to admit that they're trying to lose weight. What are the chosen strategies? Well, the list is endless, but here are a few: cleansers, rapid weight loss in 20 days, drink more water, drink black coffee, eat spicy foods, eating diet foods, take weight loss pills, eat whole foods, chew slowly, cook with various oils, and taking laxatives.

Very few of these strategies have been actually examined in well controlled research studies using human participants. The reason for this is clear. For a researcher in any country to conduct a study on humans, it must be approved by research conduct committees, who's primary focus is to protect participants against potential harm from the study. I only assume that extreme weight loss diets are never studied because they present undo harm to the research participants. For example, I cannot locate a single study where laxatives, diuretics, extreme starvation, or cleansers were evaluated for their effectiveness on weight loss. The reason is that these approaches are unhealthy, and most likely would never receive study approval because of the safety concerns.

Throughout this short journey, I will present to you the results of many research studies. For example, the National Institute on Health (NIH) funded a study to compare the Atkins, Ornish, Zone, and LEARN diets on weight loss among overweight women [3]. The researchers recruited 311, overweight, non-diabetic, and premenopausal women, and assigned them to one of the weight loss strategies. Subjects received weekly dietary instructions for two months, and then were followed up with 10 months later, for a total of 12 months. Average weight loss at 12 months for each diet were as follows: Atkins = -9.68 lbs.; Ornish = -4.84 lbs.; Zone = -3.52 lbs., and LEARN = -5.72 lbs. Weight loss among participants in the Atkins diet was statistically greater than the three other dietary strategies. This study was beautifully balanced, and the number of calories ingested between all groups was not different, meaning that participants consumed a similar number of calories in each group. As many know, the Atkins diet is a high protein, low carbohydrate strategy for weight loss, and this study established the effectiveness of consuming high protein compared to other more traditional weight loss strategies, such as low fat. In addition, the researchers reported no adverse metabolic effects such as an increase in triglycerides or blood sugar. In fact, the participants in the Atkins group demonstrated lower triglycerides, blood glucose, and also blood pressure. An important comment was made by the researchers, in which they stated their uncertainty if the weight loss was more influenced by the high protein or low carbohydrate intake among the Atkins group. It has since been determined (through well controlled studies) that the high protein strategy drives weight loss and not the low carbohydrate [4]. I will discuss this statement in more detail in Chapter 3.

You're probably asking, why shouldn't I simply eat a high protein, low carb diet? You absolutely can, and some, but not all research supports it. However, weight loss researchers have commented that it is futile to expect overweight humans to consistently consume a low carbohydrate diet [5]. In this booklet, I will present dietary strategies that may help you in your weight loss goals. Within each of these strategies, the consumption of a higher protein diet supports greater weight loss, and I make this comment throughout the manual.

I have decided to keep the cover to this manual very plain and indistinguishable. Losing weight doesn't need to be flashy, just effective. Plus, I truly believe that deciding to lose weight is a humbling moment as you've come to the conclusion that you may not be as healthy as you once were. This is a powerful decision, and you shouldn't be exposed to other's judgment.

The overall goal, is to empower you with both knowledge and strategy for losing and maintaining weight loss. I purposely designed this publication as a booklet, pocketbook, or for your tablet or smart phone device, and not to be a hard-bound text book style. My hope is that it becomes your go to manual for developing a weight loss program. I am also happy to answer any questions you may have.

My role in your weight loss journey

Throughout my education, teaching, and research, a common theme is weight loss. Discussions commonly take place among colleagues, along with undergraduate and graduate students in regards to weight loss strategies. In our exercise laboratory, we routinely measure markers of weight management, which include body composition, resting metabolic rate, blood panels, along with many cardiovascular and skeletal muscle fitness indicators. We conduct these tests among research participants, community members, and student-athletes to assist them in developing weight loss plans. We use sound practice when assisting people with weight management, which comprises making precise measurements and using science-based weight loss strategies.

I have recently developed concerns in regard to the weight loss strategies currently being advertised. Most have no research support and appear gimmicky and potentially unhealthy. My role in your weight loss journey is to present and interpret the results of well controlled research studies. In science, this is termed bench to bedside, or in other words, from research to practice. Throughout, I will highlight concerns and gaps in the knowledge. For example, most weight loss studies are less than one year in length. So, the safety of maintaining various weight loss strategies over time is concerning, and I will voice this as we move forward. As you may have already noticed, my strength is not in telling you an elegant story or attempting to entertain you. My students will most likely tell you the same; however, my intention is for you to learn and then practice what you've learned, and ultimately achieve your weight loss goals.

I am not a registered dietician, and not qualified to prescribe a diet to you; however, I have the education and training to discuss weight loss with you. I will simply detail effective weight loss strategies and provide you a framework to implement them into your life.

The takeaway

I've stated that my goal is for you to learn about weight loss strategies and then implement them into your life. I will discuss three strategies in this initial version of the manual:

1. Balance daily calorie restriction

2. Meal timing

3. Alternate day fasting

Each of these have research evidence to support their effect on weight loss. Some have more support than others (I will mention), but all appear to be effective. The next two chapters provide education regarding weight loss and dietary considerations and are intended to simply inform you. If you want to get right to the weight loss strategies then skip to section 2.

Chapter 2. Weight gain and loss

I'm not going to waste your time by reporting on overweight and obesity trends across the globe. We all know it is the number one health concern because excess body fat is linked to almost every disease state. In this section, I will briefly explain what occurs when body fat is gained and lost.

Weight gain

Weight gain can come from two main sources. The first is from increased muscle mass, or lean body mass through resistance exercise. This type of weight gain is good as muscle is highly metabolically active tissue and increasing lean mass can increase metabolic rate.

Second is weight gain from increased fat mass, or adipose tissue. This occurs when calorie intake exceeds energy expenditure, and results in an increase synthesis of adipose tissue leading to storage of energy sources. One pound of fat has an estimated calorie value of 3,500 calories, so consuming 3,500 calories over your energy expenditure leads to 1 pound of fat and can be stored throughout the body. We are all born with a certain number of fat cells, and during weight gain fat cells increase in both size and number. A normal weight person may have 30 billion fat cells compared to an overweight person who has over 100 billion fat cells [6]. Weight gain doesn't occur in a day or even a week but is commonly a residual process.

For example, let's assume that a 30-year-old man weighs 169 lbs., and has an average metabolic rate of 2,000 calories per day. This means, he burns about 2,000 calories per day, so he needs to eat 2,000 calories per day to maintain his current weight of 169 lbs. Now, if this person simply consumes 2,100 calories each day, he will have a weekly overage of 700 calories (7 days x 100 calorie overage). Over the course of a month this will be 2,800 calories (700 calories x 4-weeks), and over the year this will be 33,600 calories (2,800 calories x 12 months). Remember, 1 pound of fat equals 3,500 calories, so this person will have gained almost 10 lbs. of fat during the year (33,600 calories ÷ 3,500 calories). This is a very simplified breakdown of weight gain, and the reason for explaining it this way is to show you that it can be a very subtle process.

Weight gain can be influenced heavily by hormones (e.g., insulin, thyroid), nervous system, behavior (e.g., social activities), psychology (e.g., stress), and host of other variables. I would be remiss not to mention these; however, to keep the discussion light, I will not go into details on these factors. The take home message here is that weight gain can sneak up on you. Suddenly you're forty years old, and twenty pounds heavier than when you were thirty.

Weight loss

The ideal weight loss scenario is shedding fat while maintaining lean, or muscle mass. However, losing both is a common consequence when one loses weight. When energy expenditure exceeds energy intake then weight loss will occur. This imbalance can happen by increasing energy expenditure (i.e., exercise), decreasing energy intake (i.e., eating less), or a combination of both.

Let's look at another example of a 40-year-old female, who weighs 190 lbs. with an estimated metabolic rate of 1,800 calories. If she eats less than 1,800 calories each day then she will be in a calorie deficit (energy expenditure > energy intake). Maintaining a deficit over the course of weeks and months leads to weight loss. If this woman decides to eat 1,300 calories per day, which is a 500-calorie deficit then her estimated weekly calorie deficit will be 3,500 calories (500 calorie deficit x 7 days). This equates to 1 lb. per week of weight loss! Researchers, and dieticians recommend a calorie deficit ranging from 250 calories to 1,000 calories per day, but to never create a daily caloric deficit greater than 1,000 calories. This is considered severe calorie restriction, which we discuss in more detail later.

In a calorie deficit scenario, your body will begin breaking down fat cells for energy usage since it is not getting enough energy from your diet. Unlike weight gain where fat cells change in both size and number, during weight loss fat cells only decrease in size. The only way to get rid of fat cells is to have them surgically removed, which is popular procedure in the field of cosmetic surgery.

In this book I teach you how to calculate your metabolic rate and how to establish a calorie deficit to promote weight loss. Again, please be aware that we are taking a rather simplified approach to weight loss; however, as you will see moving forward, that **the most important factor in a weight loss plan is creating a calorie deficit.**

Where does the fat go during weight loss? The answer to this question may be surprising to you. When a molecule of fat is metabolized in the body it is broken down to carbon dioxide (CO_2), water (H_2O), and of course energy. The CO_2 is released by the lung via exhalation; the formed water is excreted through urine, sweat, tears, and breath; the energy produced is used by the body for various physiological processes. Researchers have calculated that when a human loses 10 kilograms (22 lbs.) of fat, they produce 28 kilograms (61.6 lbs.) of CO_2 and 11 kilograms (24.2 lbs.) of H_2O. So, the lung is considered the primary organ for excretion of fat, and weight loss! However, this doesn't mean that you will lose more weight if you hyperventilate all day long (you will most likely pass out)!

Chapter 3. Diet considerations

Calorie deficits

The most important aspect of a weight loss strategy is to create caloric deficit, and to sustain this calorie deficit for weeks on end [8]. For example, if you cut 500 calories per day, and sustain this for a week then you will lose approximately one pound per week. You see, one pound of fat mass is equal to 3,500 calories and cutting 500 calories daily for seven days equates to a weekly deficit of 3,500 calories, or 1 pound of fat. This approach to weight loss is moderate and sustainable, and recommended by the U.S. National Institute of Health [9]. More severe approaches are to cut > 1,000 calories per day (>2 lbs. per week), which is much harder to sustain, and may present safety concerns. See table 1 to determine daily calorie deficits and estimated overall weight loss at 26 weeks.

Table 3.1. Weight loss deficits

Weight loss	Daily deficit (calories)	Weekly deficit (calories)	Estimated 26-week weight loss
Mild = 0.5lbs per week	250	1,750	13 lbs.
Moderate = 1lb per week	500	3,500	26 lbs.
High = 1.5lb per week	750	5,250	39 lbs.
Severe > 2lb per week	1000	7000	52 lbs.

Now, to establish the number of calories that one should be eating to create a weekly calorie deficit, one must first calculate their **total energy expenditure (TEE),** which is the number of calories that the body burns during the day, and for simplification, we can refer to this as **metabolic rate**. In our research lab, we can accurately measure this value; however, equations have been developed to estimate TEE. These equations take into account age, sex, current body weight, and height[10]. Physical activity (PA) is also factored into the calculation for TEE, or metabolic rate. The equations for men and women over the age of 19 are shown below (Table 3.2; Eq. 3.1, 3.2) [10].

Creating a calorie deficit each day or week is the most important factor for weight loss! You must burn more than you ingest.

Table 3.2. Total energy expenditure calculations for men and women.

Eq.3.1. Men	TEE or metabolic rate = PA x [(4.5454 x weight in lbs.) + (15.875 x height inches) – (5 x age) +5]
Eq.3.2. Women	TEE or metabolic rate = PA x [(4.5454 x weight in lbs.) + (15.875 x height inches) – (5 x age) – 161]

To determine your physical activity factor (PA), use table 3.3. Those who do not consistently exercise and do not have a physically demanding job should select a factor of 1.0. Men will select 1.13 and women 1.12 if consistently performing light exercise or have a slightly physical occupation. The factor selected will be used in the formulas in figure 3.1 in place of the "PA".

Table 3.3. Physical activity (PA) factor

Level	Male	Female
Sedentary – no daily exercise, desk job	1.0	1.0
Light – walking, some physical nature to occupation	1.13	1.12
Moderate – exercise 3-4 times per week for 30-60 minutes. Physical occupation	1.25	1.27
Very active – heavy exercise 7 times per week. Highly physical job (wildland firefighting, heavy construction)	1.48	1.45

Let's practice the calculation for a 5'4" (64 inches), 50-year-old female, who weighs 175 lbs. We will also assume that she is sedentary, so select a physical activity factor of 1.0. I calculated her TEE or metabolic rate to be ~1,400 calories (using Eq. 3.2, table 3.2). I want to be clear that this value represents the number of calories required to maintain current body weight and is also the value used to set a calorie deficit goal. If a person consumes less calories than their metabolic rate then an energy deficit will occur and will drive weight loss.

Using our 50-year-old example, if this woman has a weight loss goal of 0.5 lbs. per week, she will need to cut 250 calories per day, or try to keep her daily caloric intake at 1,150 calories (1,150 – 250). I hope you are able to follow as you will be making these calculations in the subsequent chapters.

Now, calculate your own metabolic rate.

My metabolic rate = ████████████████ calories

In later chapters we will review ideal caloric restriction goals based on your current metabolic rate. At this point, I want to discuss a very important topic in regards to weight loss and metabolism. When someone loses weight, they are losing body tissue, which is commonly both fat and muscle. The loss of body mass causes a decrease in metabolic rate because you now have less metabolically active tissue. For example, in a 12-week weight loss study among men, the participants lost between 18-20 lbs [11]. Before the study began, the average metabolic rate among the men was 1,911 calories per day, and after weight loss their metabolic rate decreased to 1,740 calories. Again, the reason for this decrease was because they lost both fat weight and some muscle weight (or lean mass). How do we interpret and apply this information? Here is one way…if the men consume substantially more than 1,740 calories on a daily basis they will regain weight. Another is that if they want to continue to lose weight then their caloric deficit must be based on the new 1,740 calories metabolic rate.

For these reasons, I suggest recalculating your metabolic rate after every 6-weeks of a weight loss program. In addition, it may benefit you to recalculate if you become substantially more physically active, or inactive. For example, if you begin attending cycling classes several times per week then you can factor this into your metabolic rate calculation.

Before moving on, I want to briefly mention that while maintaining a caloric deficit is a major key to a weight loss strategy, other factors play a role in the amount of weight that is lost. These may include: 1. The composition of the meal (e.g., amount of protein, carbohydrate, and fat), which we will discuss later; 2. One's initial body weight. Those who weigh more tend to lose more weight during short-term weight loss (12-26 weeks); 3. Age. The targeted weight loss strategies may be more or less effective because of the aging process; 4. The amount of exercise, which we will discuss in Chapter 7; and 5. Genetics. Some people are very successful in achieving their weight loss goals, while others do not have the same positive results despite following a rigid weight loss strategy. In science, these participants are called responders, and non-responders, respectively. It is very difficult to identify the reasons for these differences, and they may be partially attributed to gene expression [12]. I'm sure we could identify several more beyond the five that I have listed. I make an attempt in this book to simplify weight loss, but as many of you know, or have experienced firsthand, that many other factors (such as those stated) can play a role.

High protein and low carbohydrate dietary strategies

The origin of the high protein low carbohydrate diet can be traced to biblical times, but the popularity escalated with the emergence of the Atkin's diet [13]. Before the Atkins craze, the approach to weight loss was reducing calories through low fat dietary options. Hence, the abundance of low fat items on grocery store shelves. Since Atkins, many dieticians have begun to prescribe a higher protein dietary strategy to those aiming to lose weight. The recommended daily allowance for protein is 0.8 grams per kilogram of body weight [14]. For a 200 lb. (90 kg.) person, this would be around 72 g. of protein per day. Most Americans consume about 15% of their diet from protein sources. Diets in which people consume 25% of their diet from protein are considered high protein diets, and commonly equate to roughly 1.6 grams of protein per kilogram body weight. Again, for our 200 lb. (90 kg.) person, this would be nearly 144 grams per day. Any diet that is higher than 35% protein, or more than 2.4 g/kg/day (about 214 g/d for our 200 lb. person) is considered an extremely high protein diet [15]. Before going further, let me say that the safety of long term (more than 12 months) high protein diets is uncertain. I will review related research on this topic next.

In the past 10-15 years researchers have aggressively studied high protein diets for weight loss. Common interventions used by weight loss researchers have been adjusting diets to 25-40% protein with 32-50% carbohydrate and 15-25% from fat (15-25%). Keep in mind that these dietary interventions all have participants consuming a low-calorie diet. For example, in a 2007 study, all participants consumed the same number of calories each day (~1,500 calories/day) for 64 weeks [16]. However, one group was asked to consume a higher protein diet (34% protein, 20% fat, 46% carbs) while a second group was asked to consume a high carbohydrate diet (17% protein, 20% fat, 64% carbs). At the end of the 64-week intervention it was shown that those subjects who maintained the high protein diet lost more weight. More specifically, those who consumed more than 88 grams of protein per day lost more weight. However, both groups did lose weight at the end of the study.

It has been shown that in well controlled weight loss studies that when a high protein diet vs. a balanced diet are compared, the weight loss results are mixed [15]. Meaning that some high protein diets result in greater weight loss while others show no differences between the groups, meaning they lose the same amount of weight [16]. For example, when a group of obese participants ate a high protein diet (25% protein, 30% fat, 45% carbs) they lost nearly 16 lbs. over 27 weeks. The high carbohydrate group (12% protein, 30% fat, 58% carbs) lost 11 lbs. in the same 27-week period [17]. Now, if we look a little deeper into these results, it was determined that those in the high protein diet consumed less overall calories. Always remember, the most important thing in a weight loss intervention is creating an energy deficit (as previously discussed), which was greater in the high protein group. This indicated that consuming a higher protein diet may lead to greater satiety (feeling of fullness), and cause overall lower food intake, which is discussed more later in the chapter [18].

In another study among obese women, a high protein group consisting of 30% protein was compared to a group on a standard protein diet of 15% protein. Both groups of women ate 1,200 calories per day over a 10-week time frame. At the end of the study the high protein group lost 14 lbs. while the standard protein group lost almost 12 lbs. Again, you can see the results were very similar [19].

As more results are being publish in regard to the added weight loss benefit of a higher protein diet it has become clearer that increasing the percentage of protein results in slightly more weight loss. The added value has been estimated at 4 additional pounds in weight loss studies [20]. This may seem marginal, but is regarded as statistically important. Now, because of the mixed results in regards to higher protein diets, I do not specifically recommend this approach for each of the weight loss strategies described in the later chapters. I do however mention that increasing the percentage of protein ingestion in each strategy may lead to greater weight loss results.

You may have heard of the ketogenic diet, or the term "living keto". This dietary approach comprises severe low carbohydrate combined with high protein and fat. A daily carbohydrate intake of 50 grams, which is extremely low, is considered a ketogenic diet, and is termed very low carbohydrate ketogenic diet (VLCKD) [21]. In review of VLCKDs, it was determined that weight loss is dependent on calorie restriction and the duration of the dietary restriction, and not dependent on the low carbohydrate composition of the diet [22]. In a handful of studies, it has been determined that short term weight loss (4-6 months) is greater when one uses a low carbohydrate dietary approach, but after 6 months weight loss is the same compared to balanced dietary strategies [22]. Because the ketogenic diet is a big lifestyle adjustment, and also because of the uncertainty of long term safety of this approach, I do not recommend the VLCKD in this book. In addition, researchers have highlighted the difficulty for people to remain compliant when assigned to a low carbohydrate diet. Meaning that people just do not enjoy drastically cutting carbohydrate.

In the next few paragraphs I will explain what is happening to your body when consuming a low carbohydrate and high protein diet, and I will also explain some theories as to why this approach may be effective during short term weight loss (less than 6 months). If you have no interest in learning, or do not have the time then skip to the next section.

When you begin a low carbohydrate diet, you will deplete your carbohydrate stores, or called glycogen stores, in the muscle and liver. Stored carbohydrate also retains water, so when it is depleted, the associated water is also lost. The early weight loss (1 week or slightly longer) may be attributed to reduced water weight.

After the stored glycogen is depleted the body will begin to rely on other energy sources to support all bodily functions. This can occur after 3-4 days of very low carbohydrate consumption (50 g/day). To support the body's energy needs, an increase rate of fat and protein metabolism will take place, and a byproduct of these sources are ketone bodies. The build-up of ketone bodies is called ketogenesis, which occurs primarily in the liver. The production of ketone bodies can then be used by tissues as a source of energy other than glucose. The ketosis is considered a normal physiological response and is differentiated from the pathological form that can be developed in type 1 diabetics by the level of ketones in the blood. In the normal state ketones reach maximal levels of 8 mmol/l with no change in the body's pH level. In type 1 diabetics, ketones can rise above 20 mmol/l leading to lowering of pH, and the potential for bodily harm. As you can see, ketosis is an active physiological response, and because of the uncertainty about the safety of this diet, I cannot suggest it to you.

When one consumes a high protein diet there appears to be some added metabolic and dietary behavior advantages that may support weight loss. I have highlighted these below with short explanations.

1. Those who consume over 25% protein in their diet report greater satiety and ultimately a reduction in appetite. This has been shown in several studies [17, 18, 23]. Have you ever consumed a can of tuna and noticed how full you feel? A can of tuna is about 120 calories but has nearly 30g of protein.
2. An increase in metabolic rate due to the higher energy cost to digest and absorb high protein meals. This may lead to an overall higher metabolic rate [24].
3. Higher protein diets may preserve metabolism, or metabolic rate during weight loss [25]. This response has yet to be adequately explained.

Meal frequency

You have probably read somewhere that increasing the number of small meals each day leads to greater weight loss. It seems that the common number is six meals per day. The logic for this approach is to keep the hunger monster at bay so that you do not over eat. Everyone has gone long periods without eating, which commonly leads to overeating. Another reason is that when you eat, you increase your metabolic rate because your body uses energy to digest and absorb foods. Consuming many meals throughout the day may help to maintain a higher metabolism over the day.

So, the question is…does meal frequency effect weight loss? A group of researchers examined all meal frequency studies since 2015, and based on all of the results determined that meal frequency was not associated with changes in body mass [26]. Meaning that there is no difference in body mass changes between consuming 1-2 meals per day or more than five. However, in further analysis, the researchers discovered that a higher number of meals was associated with a greater decrease in body fat percentage. This may indicate that more fat mass is being lost and lean body mass is being preserved. However, this result was largely based on one study, so uncertainty remains about whether or not meal frequency is an effective weight loss strategy [27]. Again, I will always remind you that maintaining a caloric deficit is the most important variable in a weight loss program. Increasing meal frequency while meeting the caloric deficit goal may help prevent hunger and may lead to greater fat loss. The jury is still out though.

Section 2. Weight loss Strategies

Three weight loss strategies will be discussed in the following chapters. These will include:

Chapter 4. Balanced daily calorie restriction (BDCR)
Chapter 5. Meal timing
Chapter 6. Alternate day fasting

In each chapter, I provide a short description and research support for the strategy, along with steps of how to implement the weight loss program into your life. Lastly, I will discuss the role of exercise in your weight loss program (Chapter 7).

Below is comparison of three dietary strategies on short term weight ranging between 12 to 24 weeks. These estimates are based on reported results from research studies. You can see that if you commit to one of the following strategies then weight loss will most likely occur.

	Balance daily calorie restriction	Meal timing	Alternate day fasting
Weight loss ranges for 12 – 24 week studies	10 – 18 lbs.	9 – 22 lbs.	6 – 16 lbs.

Results may vary for each person (both more or less weight loss).

Chapter 4. Evidence-based weight loss strategy one: balanced daily calorie restriction (BDCR)

Alright, let's get to it. The plan is to present several evidence-based weight loss strategies that you can install into your life. The first is creating a calorie restriction each day, and balancing the calorie cut across each meal. We will term this balanced daily calorie restriction (BDCR). Commonly studied calorie restriction diets comprise a 25% energy reduction [28]. Using a 2,000-calorie example, this would be reducing daily intake to 1,500 calories per day, and the calorie restriction distributed across each meal. Let's break it down a little more.

Step 1. Calculate daily metabolic rate (Eqs. 3.1 and 3.2, table 3.2) = 2,000.

Step 2. Calorie intake goal (25% reduction) = 1,500 calories.

Step 3. The 1,500-calorie diet will be distributed across each meal. If you eat three meals per day, then each will be 500 calories.

Another common method for determining the amount of calorie restriction is basing it on the weekly weight loss goals. If you recall from Chapter 3, table 3.1, you can estimate your weekly weight loss by calculating a daily caloric deficit. The deficit is also based on subtracting these calories from your metabolic rate calculation. For example, if the goal is to lose 1.5 lbs. per week then 750 calories must be cut from your daily diet. Using the hypothetical 2,000 calorie metabolic rate, the estimated number of calories to eat each day is 1,250. Consuming this daily amount will promote a 1.5 lbs. per week weight loss. Similar to the 25% reduction discussed above, the 1,250 calories are distributed across each of the meals, regardless of meal frequency.

The initial studies exploring calorie restriction used the BDCR approach. In a well-controlled study, a group of researchers had overweight participants consume a 25% reduction diet for 6 months [28]. The meal compositions were balanced with less than 30% fat, which is the recommendation from the American Heart Association [29]. ***At the end of the six-month study time frame, the participants lost 10% of their body weight, or an average of nearly 18 lbs.*** In addition, participants showed a decrease in fasting insulin, which is an important metabolic measure. The results of this study demonstrate the effectiveness of a calorie restriction diet of 25% daily reduction.

Similar results have been reported when weekly calories are cut by a standard number to achieve weekly weight loss goals as opposed to the 25% reduction. In a 2017 study, obese Latino men and women were asked to reduce their daily calorie intake by 500 calories, which estimates weekly weight loss at 1 pound (see Chapter 3, table 3.1) [19]. *__The study was 6 months in length and the participants lost between 11-15 lbs.__* You may be wondering why they didn't lose more weight? When looking a little closer, it was reported that nearly twenty-five percent of the participants did not follow the diet, which lowered the average weight loss among the group. *However, __the participants who followed the calorie restriction during the diet lost over 20 lbs.!__*

Let's take a look at another very interesting study. In this one, researchers separated overweight women into a high protein low-carbohydrate or low-fat calorie restriction diet for six months [30]. Both groups, reduced intake by 450 calories each day, or roughly 26% reduction in nutrient intake. Both groups ingested roughly 1,200 calories per day. Let me explain the composition of the high protein and low-fat diets in this study. The high protein group consumed roughly 23% of their diet from carbohydrate, 27% from protein, and 52% from fat. Now, in the low-fat group the participants consumed roughly 54% carbohydrate, 18% protein, and 28% fat during the 6-month trial. *__The participants in the high protein group lost nearly 20 lbs. at the end of 6-months while the low-fat group lost roughly 9 lbs.__* While both groups lost weight, you can see the higher protein approach was more effective. Again, this highlights the benefit of a higher proportion of protein in the diet composition of a weight loss strategy. However, it is important to mention that this study was only 6 months in duration.

Another very important discussion point is the level of calorie restriction. There have been several studies in which overweight or obese participants were put on medically supervised very low-calorie diets (VLCD) that ranged from 420 – 800 calories per day [31, 32]. These are considered extreme weight loss strategies, which require attentive medical supervision, and I do not recommend unless you are under the care of a physician and dietician. In addition, this level of calorie restriction is nearly impossible for participants to maintain, and commonly result in weight regain. Researchers in the mid-90s compared a VLCD (420 calories per day) to a moderate 25% reduction calorie restriction diet (1,200 calories per day) among obese women. The women in both groups were tracked over an entire year. *At mid-year (6 months), the women in the VLCD lost more weight, nearly 46 lbs. compared to the 25% reduction group, who lost 24 lbs*. However, *over the next 6 months, the women in the VLCD re-gained weight, and by the end of the year weight loss for both groups ranged from 20-22 lbs. overall* [31].

The bulk of BDCR studies have ranged from 4 to 24 weeks in length and have produced average weight loss of 5-8%. *For a 250 lb. person, the weight loss would be 12-20 lbs*. These results are very promising, especially for short term weight loss goals. In accordance with the weight loss in BDCR studies, participants routinely demonstrate improvements in important markers of metabolic function such as blood glucose, A1c, and insulin sensitivity [33, 34].

Developing the strategy

To develop an effective BDCR strategy, you must be organized and pay attention to detail. It appears from the research using either a calorie restriction of 25% or using a daily 500-750 calorie deficit (1 to 1.5 lbs. per week) are both effective and sustainable, so I recommend these levels of restriction if you choose this weight loss approach. Here are the steps to adequately develop the BDCR diet. I have first provided an example of how to develop a 25% reduction BDCR dietary strategy then you can calculate your own.

Example:
Female
45 years old
Non-active (PA = 1, from table 3.3)
Body weight: 182 lbs.
Height: 64 inches (5 feet, 4 inches)

Step 1. Metabolic rate = 1,632 calories per day. This was determined based on gender, age, and current weight. Also factored in is the person's daily activity level (see Eq. 3.2).

Step 2a. Weight loss goal = 25% daily calorie reduction (1,632 calories x .25% = 408 calories).

Step 2b. Daily calorie restriction = 408 calories.

Step 3. Daily calorie intake = 1,632 calories – 408 calories = 1,224 calories per day.

The number of calories this person should eat each day to lose weight

Step 4. Per meal energy intake = 1,224 / # of meals.

1,224 / 4 meals = 306 calories per meal (note, I chose 4 meals for this example).

The calorie intake (i.e., 1,224 calories) is balanced across the entire day by dividing the number of meals by the targeted number of calories

Below is a diet plan for this example.

Table 4.1. food log for BDCR

Food description	Nutrient breakdown (estimations)	Calories
Meal 1 = 306 calories goal (7am)		
Egg white sandwich from McDonalds	7g fat, 18g pro, 27g cho	250
Orange (1 ct)	0g fat, 1g pro, 11g cho	45
Coffee (with cream)	NA	0
	Total	295
Meal 2 = 306 calories goal (11am)		
Small turkey sandwich (wheat bread, lettuce, tomato, mustard)	6g fat, 26g pro, 33g cho	290
Diet Coke or water or both	NA	0
	Total	290
Meal 3 = 306 calories goal (3pm)		
Protein supplement bar	8g fat, 20g pro, 30g cho	270
	Total	270
Meal 4 = 306 calories goal (7pm)		
Chicken breast grilled (~224 grams)	6g fat, 46g pro, 0 cho	220
Green beans 1 cup	0g fat, 1g pro, 6g cho	30
Glass of white wine (6.8 oz)	0g fat, .1 pro, 2.7g cho	144
	Total	394
Daily totals	**27g fat, 112g pro, 109g cho**	**1,249**

g-grams, pro-protein, cho-carbohydrate. Total fat calories = 243, total protein calories = 448, and total carbohydrate calories = 436. Calorie totals may not equal nutrient totals due to estimations

Another strategy is to base calorie restriction on achieving weekly weight loss goals, according to Chapter 3, table 3.1. Again, a daily deficit of 500-750 calories is effective and sustainable.

Using the same 45-year-old example from above (see figure 4.1):

Step 1. Metabolic rate = 1,632 calories per day.

Step 2a. Weight loss goal = 1.5 lbs. per week loss (I chose 1.5 lbs. for this example).

<u>Step 2b</u>. Daily calorie restriction = 750 calories (Table 3.1).

> Cutting 750 calories per day will result in an estimated 1.5 lbs. weight loss per week (see table 3.1).

<u>Step 3.</u> Daily calorie intake = 1,632 calories − 750 calories = 882 calories per day.

> The number of calories this person should eat each day to lose weight

<u>Step 4</u>. Per meal energy intake = 882 / # of meals.
   882 / 3 meals = 277 calories per meal (note, I chose 3 meals for this example), and apply to the diet log.

I hope you can see how simple these calculations are for establishing the deficits. You must decide which calorie restriction number works for you. If you're feeling extremely hungry then increase calorie intake; and, conversely if you're feeling satisfied then maybe try to cut a little more.

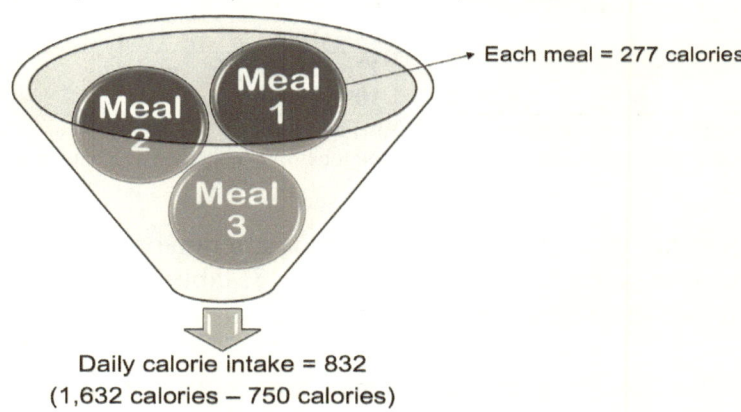

e 1.5 lbs. per week for a person with a TEE = 1,632 calories

Each meal = 277 calories

Meal 1
Meal 2
Meal 3

Daily calorie intake = 832
(1,632 calories − 750 calories)

Figure 4.1. BDCR based on weight loss per week. For this example, the calculated TEE is 1,632 calories, and the person's goal is to lose 1.5 lbs. per week. This will require a daily deficit of 750 calories per day. The deficit is balanced across 3 meals all of which are 277 calories. TEE − total energy expenditure.

When viewing the food log in table 4.1, you may be wondering about including McDonalds (meal 1) or a glass of wine (meal 4). I understand that meal planning is difficult, and you can still make good dietary decisions when eating out. Also, if you enjoy a cocktail then no problem, just factor the additional calories into the plan. Remember, weight loss is the most dependent on creating a calorie deficit! If consuming fast food or a glass of wine still allows you to maintain a calorie deficit then weight loss will occur! Just don't make it a habit.

Also, the amount of detail that you put into your food log is up to you. Personally, I only pay attention to the calorie value as listing nutrients can be exhausting. Fortunately, several nutrition tracking websites are available that have thousands of food items in their databases and will calculate the nutrient information for you (see appendix B).

Below I have provided the steps below for you to complete for developing a BDCR strategy. I have greyed out the areas for you to complete the calculations.

Step 1. Calculate your metabolic rate (enter the information below)

Age: _____.

Height (ht.): _____ in.

Body weight (wt.): _____ lbs.

Perform the calculation using equations below and your PA from table 4.2.

| Men | TEE or metabolic rate = PA x [(4.5454 x weight in lbs.) + (15.875 x height inches) – (5 x age) +5] |
| Women | TEE or metabolic rate = PA x [(4.5454 x weight in lbs.) + (15.875 x height inches) – (5 x age) – 161] |

Table 4.2. Physical activity (PA) factor

Level	Male	Female
Sedentary – no daily exercise, desk job	1.0	1.0
Light – walking, some physical nature to occupation	1.13	1.12
Moderate – exercise 3-4 times per week for 30-60 minutes. Physical occupation	1.25	1.27
Very active – heavy exercise 7 times per week. Highly physical job (wildland firefighting, heavy construction)	1.48	1.45

Your calculated TEE or metabolic rate = _____ calories per day.

Remember, this is your calculated metabolic rate

Step 2a. Weight loss goal: Choose your goal (select below).
Daily 25% reduction or weekly weight loss strategy (1 to 1.5 lbs. per week).

Step 2b. Daily calorie restriction.
Calculate the number of calories to consume based on a 25% restriction.

TEE or metabolic rate (from step 1) x .25 = _____ 25% reduction daily reduction.

Or

Determine the number of calories to consume based on weekly weight loss strategy, recommend either 500 or 750 calorie reduction each day.

_____ = daily calorie reduction.
(select 500 - 750 calories)

Step 3. Calculate the number of calories to eat based on weekly weight loss goal (Chapter 3, Table 3.1).

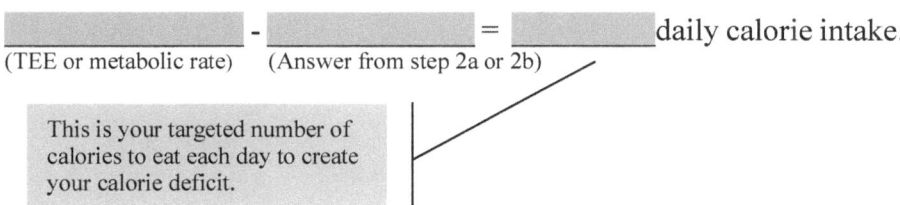

_____ - _____ = _____ daily calorie intake.
(TEE or metabolic rate)   (Answer from step 2a or 2b)

This is your targeted number of
calories to eat each day to create
your calorie deficit.

Step 4. Distribute this reduction across your meal frequency or pattern.

The daily calorie intake value is your new calorie intake target. You will distribute this across your day. In the food log table below, I have made space for 4 meals; however, the number is up to you. See appendix D for more blank food log sheets.

Table 4.3. Blank food log for BDCR

Food description	Nutrient breakdown (estimations)	Calories
Meal 1 = _____ calories goal (7am)		
	Total	**=**
Meal 2 = _____ calories goal (11am)		
	Total	**=**
Meal 3 = _____ calories goal (3pm)		
	Total	**=**
Meal 4 = _____ calories goal (7pm)		
	Total	**=**
Daily total		**=**

Step 5. Readjust diet based on weight loss.

I suggest repeating steps 1-4 every 6-weeks. As you lose weight, your metabolic rate will decrease, so to maintain weight loss you will need to adjust your calorie deficit goal. Once you achieve your weight loss goals, I suggest calculating your new metabolic rate to sustain your weight loss goals. If you resort back to your original diet or lifestyle, you will then regain your weight.

Pros and cons

The balanced daily calorie restriction (BDCR) approach to weight loss has proven to be an effective strategy. Participants in weight loss studies have consistently lost weight. The reason is that you're creating a daily negative energy balance, which favors weight loss. As with any dietary strategy, there are both pros and cons. I list these in table 4.4.

Table 4.4. BDCR pros and cons.

Pros	Cons
A 25% reduction is sustainable for at least a year.	Longer term effect of BDCR is unknown. One known longitudinal (4 years) study shows that weight regain does occur [5].
In research studies, a 25% reduction leads to weight loss of 10 to 18 lbs. at 6 months [28, 35], and nearly 20 lbs. at 12 months [31].	Higher caloric deficits will lead to greater weight loss, but difficult to sustain.
Daily calorie restriction of 500 calorie leads to weight loss of 11 to 20 lbs. over a short-term period (<6 months).	Some studies have reported poor adherence. Meaning that some dieters have trouble with the consistency of the daily balanced calorie restriction strategy
Higher percentage of protein in BDCR diet leads to greater weight loss. 25%-35% protein is recommended [4, 5].	Very low-calorie diets, or severe calorie restriction (~800 calories/day) are not recommended. This approach must be under the supervision of a physician.
Body fat and body mass index decrease.	Common to lose muscle mass (see the Role of Exercise section below).
Improvement in markers of metabolism (e.g., blood glucose, insulin, A1c) [34].	Must have a dietary plan and be organized. This may lead to the inability to sustain the BDCR diet.

Chapter 5. Evidence-based weight loss strategy two: meal timing strategy

I'm sure you know someone (maybe yourself) who skips breakfast, or eats very light in morning, and then may go on to consume a large lunch and/or dinner. If you remember, the original Slim Fast diet was in many ways based on this approach. People were encouraged to drink a Slim Fast shake for breakfast and lunch, and then prepare their own dinner. This approach is designed to achieve a daily calorie deficit; however, the amount of food consumed across each meal is different. Similar to the Slim Fast example, in the meal timing strategy a person consumes a low-calorie breakfast, typically around 250 calories, and then a mid-sized lunch (roughly 500 calories), and finally, a large sized dinner (750 calories). This equates to 1,500 calories per day, similar to the 25% calorie restriction diet discussed in chapter 4. In addition, the pattern of meal timing can be reversed. In this approach, someone will consume a large breakfast (~750 calories), a medium-sized lunch (~500 calories), and a small dinner (~250 calories).

Let's review some well controlled research studies on meal timing. In a study published in 2013, a group of researchers compared two different meal timing strategies among obese women over a 12-week period [36]. The participants in the study either consumed a high breakfast (700 calories), medium lunch (500 calories), and small dinner (200 calories); or the reversed, a small breakfast (200 calories), medium lunch (500 calories), and high dinner (700 calories). Both meal timing strategies were matched for calorie intake (approximately 1,400 calories), so participants ate the same amount of food. ***The high breakfast group lost more weight with nearly an 11% (about 20 lbs.) reduction in weight, while the high dinner lost 4% (about 9 lbs.) body weight.*** This demonstrates that consuming a larger proportion of your calories in the early part of the day leads to greater weight loss, but the reverse strategy (high dinner) also leads to weight loss, just not as much. Another important finding of this study was that the women in both groups had reductions in important markers of metabolic health, including in triglycerides, glucose, and insulin [37]. Again, we can interpret these results to mean that both meal timing strategies are effective; however, if you adopt this approach, you may see better weight loss results following the high breakfast pattern.

In a similar study among a group of 420 overweight participants it was demonstrated that those who were early eaters lost more weight than late eaters after a 20-week weight loss diet [38]. ***The early eaters lost nearly 22 lbs. while the late eaters lost roughly 17 lbs. Again, both groups lost weight, but eating early appears to be slightly more effective.*** This study was slightly different as it was conducted among a Mediterranean population, where lunch is traditionally the largest meal of the day. So, the group that was considered early eaters, commonly consumed lunch early in the day, and followed it with an early, and lighter dinner. The later eaters tended to consume their lunch later in the day, which led to a later dinner as well.

It is important to mention that the weight loss in the meal timing strategy is still based on creating a caloric deficit across the day, but the pattern of food intake is adjusted. The calorie reduction can be easily calculated and then applied across each meal. The approach that has been used in studies is to set the light meal at 14% of calorie goal; the medium meal at 35% of the calorie goal; and the large meal at 51% of calorie goal. I will be honest, I have subscribed to the meal timing strategy for the past 10 years, in which I typically consume a light breakfast and lunch and have a larger dinner. For me, eating large meals for breakfast or lunch doesn't work well for my schedule, so it is partially due to convenience. Sometimes I do find myself excessively hungry when dinner time arrives, which may lead to slight overeating. My hope is that I created enough of an energy deficit during the day that dinner can't make up the difference.

Similar to the BDCR diet, eating a higher protein diet at each meal also leads to greater weight loss. For example, those who consumed nearly 41% of their calories at each meal from protein, regardless of meal timing strategy, lost more weight [39].

Developing the strategy

The weight loss strategy should begin with calculating your daily metabolic rate, or the number of calories your body requires each day. The next step is deciding your weight loss goal and distributing the amount across the day. Let's take a look, and then you can make your own calculations.

Example:
Male
48 years old
Non-active (sedentary)
Body weight: 250lbs
Height: 72 inches (6 feet tall)

Step 1. Metabolic rate = 2,044 calories per day. This was determined based on gender, age, and current weight. Also factored in is the person's daily activity level (Chapter 3, Eq. 3.1).

Step 2. Weight loss goal = 1.5 pounds per week, or a reduction in 750 calories per day (Chapter 3, Table 3.1). I chose 1.5 lbs. for this example.

Step 3. Daily calorie intake goal = 1,294 calories per day (2,044 – 750) to achieve weight loss goal.

The number of calories this person should eat each day to lose weight

Step 4. Select meal timing strategy = large breakfast (note: I chose large breakfast for this example).

Breakfast goal is 51% of diet = 659 calories (1,294 x .51).
Lunch goal is 35% of diet = 453 calories (1,294 x .35).
Dinner goal is 14% of diet = 181 calories (1,294 x .14).

Choose your meal timing strategy, either high breakfast or high dinner.

Below is a diet plan for this example.

Table 5.1. Food log example for high breakfast meal timing strategy

Food description	Nutrient breakdown (estimations)	Calories
Breakfast = 703 calories goal (7am)		
2 eggs	10g fat, 12g pro, 1.2g cho	156
Sausage links (2 ct)	19g fat, 6g pro, 1g cho	200
Toast (2 slices wheat)	2g fat, 4g pro, 30g cho	154
Banana medium size (1 ct)	.4g fat, 1.3g pro, 27g cho	105
Coffee (with cream)	NA	0
	Total	615
Lunch = 483 calories goal (12pm)		
Turkey sandwich (wheat bread, cheddar cheese, mustard)	10g fat, 36 pro, 33g cho	360
Snack bag potato chips	7g fat, 2g pro, 2g cho	142
Diet soda or no calorie drink	NA	0
	Total	502
Dinner = 193 calories goal (6pm)		
Clam chowder soup (light)	6 fat, 6g pro, 30g cho	200
	Total	200
Daily totals	**54g fat, 67g pro, 124g cho**	**1,317**

g-grams, pro-protein, cho-carbohydrate. Total fat calories = 486, total protein calories = 268, and total carbohydrate calories = 496. Calorie totals may not equal nutrient totals due to estimations.

The dietary example in table 5.1 is 21% protein, which is considered a slightly higher protein diet than the typical 15%. If this person maintained a similar diet to this they would lose roughly 1.5 lbs. per week. You can see that the total for this particular day is slightly higher than calorie goal (1,294 calories vs. 1,317 calories). Every 6-weeks, the person should re-evaluate their metabolic rate, and adjust the diet accordingly. If you do not have the time to develop the diet plan then another strategy is to eat until you are satisfied at breakfast and then try to restrict (eat very little) throughout the rest of the day. If you choose the high dinner meal timing strategy then try to restrict yourself during breakfast and lunch, and then eat until you feel satisfied at dinner. These strategies will get you into the meal timing routine, and you can monitor your weight loss for effectiveness.

To lose 1.5 lbs. per week for a person with a TEE = 2,044 calories

High breakfast strategy

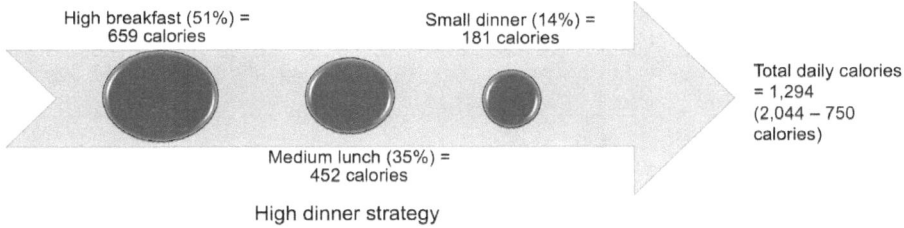

High breakfast (51%) = 659 calories

Small dinner (14%) = 181 calories

Total daily calories = 1,294 (2,044 – 750 calories)

Medium lunch (35%) = 452 calories

High dinner strategy

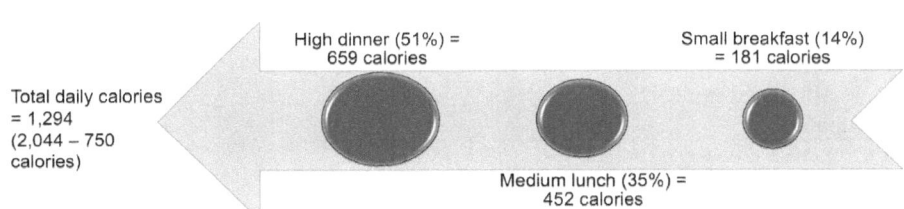

High dinner (51%) = 659 calories

Small breakfast (14%) = 181 calories

Total daily calories = 1,294 (2,044 – 750 calories)

Medium lunch (35%) = 452 calories

Figure 5.1. Meal timing strategy. In this example the person has an estimated metabolic rate of 2,044 calories, and aims to lose 1.5 lbs. per week, which is creating a 750 daily calorie deficit. Top arrow represents the high breakfast strategy with 51% calories at breakfast, 35% at lunch, and 14% at dinner. Bottom arrow represents high dinner strategy with 14% of calories consumed at breakfast, 35% at lunch, and 51% at dinner. Both strategies have been shown to be effective for weight loss.

Use the steps below to calculate your own meal timing strategy using either high breakfast, or high dinner. I have greyed out the areas for you to complete the calculations.

Step 1. Calculate metabolic rate.

Age: _____.

Height: _____ in.

Body weight: _____ lbs.

Perform the calculation using the equations below and your PA from table 5.2.

Eq.3.1. Men	TEE or metabolic rate = PA x [(4.5454 x weight in lbs.) + (15.875 x height inches) – (5 x age) +5]
Eq.3.2. Women	TEE or metabolic rate = PA x [(4.5454 x weight in lbs.) + (15.875 x height inches) – (5 x age) – 161]

Table 5.2. Physical activity (PA) factor

Level	Male	Female
Sedentary – no daily exercise, desk job	1.0	1.0
Light – walking, some physical nature to occupation	1.13	1.12
Moderate – exercise 3-4 times per week for 30-60 minutes. Physical occupation	1.25	1.27
Very active – heavy exercise 7 times per week. Highly physical job (wildland firefighting, heavy construction)	1.48	1.45

Your calculated TEE or metabolic rate = _____ calories per day.

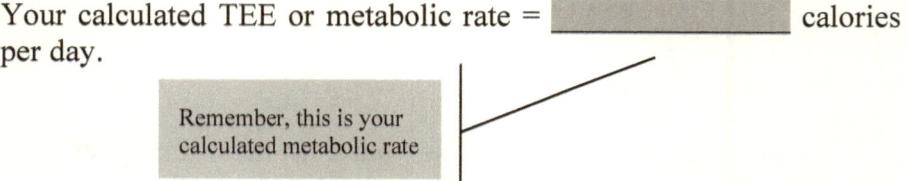

Remember, this is your calculated metabolic rate

Step 2. Determine weight loss goal per week.

500 daily calorie reduction = 1 lb. per week.
750 daily calorie reduction = 1.5 lbs. per week.

Step 3. Daily calorie intake.

_____ - _____ = _____ daily calorie intake.
(TEE or metabolic rate)   (Answer from step 2)

38

Step 4. Determine meal timing strategy.

High breakfast meal timing strategy.

Breakfast, 51% of calories = ______________ calories (answer from step 3 x .51).

Lunch, 35% of calories = ______________ calories (answer from step 3 x .35).

Dinner, 14% of calories = ______________ calories (answer from step 3 x .14).

High dinner meal timing strategy.

Breakfast, 14% of calories = ______________ calories (answer from step 3 x .14).

Lunch, 35% of calories = ______________ calories (answer from step 3 x .35).

Dinner, 51% of calories = ______________ calories (answer from step 3 x .51).

Step 5. Develop a tentative meal plan.

Nutrition calculators are available online to assist you designing your diet. It is challenging to create and follow a daily food diet. I suggest creating an example of the types and amounts of food you will be able to eat in each meal timing strategy. This will inform you about various foods that you may want to include. See appendix E for additional blank food logs.

Table 5.3. Blank food log for meal timing strategy

Food description	Nutrient breakdown (estimations)	Calories
Breakfast = _____ calories goal		
	Total	
Lunch = _____ calories goal		
	Total	
Dinner = _____ calories goal		
	Total	
Daily totals		

Step 6. Readjust diet based on weight loss.

I suggest repeating steps 1-4 every 6-weeks. As you lose weight, your metabolic rate will decrease, so to maintain weight loss you will need to adjust your meal timing calorie goals. Once you achieve your weight loss goals, I suggest calculating your new metabolic rate to sustain your weight loss goals.

Pros and cons

The advantages and disadvantages of the meal timing strategy are presented in table 5.4. This approach to weight loss may be easier to implement because it requires less structure than the BDCR strategy. A good starting point is to restrict yourself in the early part of the day and eat to fullness in the evening. Conversely, eat until you are satisfied in the morning, and try to restrict yourself throughout the day. It may also be more manageable to implement during the work week as the structure of meal timing may fit your weekday schedule. Try to maintain through the weekend, but you may need flexibility due to weekend engagements (e.g., social events).

Table 5.4. Pros and cons for meal timing strategy

Pros	Cons
Effective for weight loss in short-term studies (12 to 20 weeks).	Longer duration (> 1 year) studies do not exist, so long-term safety and sustainability are unknown.
Weight loss ranges between 9 to 22 lbs.	Common to lose muscle mass (see the Role of Exercise section below).
Consuming the majority of calories earlier in the day is more effective for weight loss.	May cause over eating if smaller meals are inadequate because of heightened feelings of hunger.
May be easier to follow than BDCR because it requires less structure and organization.	Adherence rates are unknown.
Restricting yourself earlier in the day may be easier because you're preoccupied with work and other chores.	
Body fat and body mass index decrease.	
Improvement in markers of metabolism (e.g., blood glucose, insulin, A1c).	

Chapter 6. Evidence-based weight loss strategy three: alternate day fasting

Similar to the meal timing approach to weight loss, the alternate day fasting strategy creates a calorie deficit through an unconventional eating pattern. Again, remember that the most important factor to drive weight loss is creating a calorie deficit (how many times have I said this now?). Alternate day fasting is creating the calorie deficit by following an energy restriction diet every other day, which are separated by "feast" days where one consumes a normal diet. For example, on Monday, Wednesday, Friday, and Sunday someone will consume roughly 500 calories for the entire day (i.e., fasting day). Then on Tuesday, Thursday, and Monday they will eat whatever they choose regardless of calorie content (i.e., feast day). The theory is that the weekly calorie deficits created during each fasting day cannot be overcome by the feast days. Several weight loss books have been published regarding the alternate day fasting dietary strategy, but it wasn't until 2013 that well controlled research studies were conducted.

The common alternate day fasting approach is to consume roughly 25% of calorie needs, or 25% of metabolic rate on the fasting days. For someone who has a metabolic rate of 2,000 calories, this would be 500 calories (2,000 calories x .25). On "feast" days one is permitted to consume food at their pleasure (or *ad libitum*). For the 2,000-calorie metabolic rate example, this person would eat whatever they choose. *In short duration studies ranging from 3 to 6 months, overweight humans have lost 3 to 7% of their body weight. This would be 6 to 14 pounds for a 200 lb. person* [40, 41]. In one of the earlier studies, fifteen overweight participants (age ~47) were recruited to participate in a 12-week alternate day fasting diet. On the fasting days they consumed 26% of their metabolic rate, which ranged between 400 to 600 calories. On feast days, the participants consumed as much food as desired. *At the end of the 12 weeks, the participants lost an average of 11.5 lbs., or nearly one pound per week* [40]. The researchers in the study were curious if participants felt satisfied, or if they were hungry during the fasting days. They discovered that throughout the 12-week trial, the participant's hunger level was fairly low, but so was their level of satisfaction. This indicates that while they weren't extremely hungry, they weren't satisfied either. Only one participant was unable to adhere to the alternate day fasting diet, which is very promising for utilization in long term weight loss.

This study led researchers to ask just this very question, is alternate day fasting sustainable as a longer-term weight loss strategy? In a 2017 study, thirty-four obese participants enrolled in a 12-month alternate day fasting study and were compared to a group of thirty-five obese participants, who were prescribed the BDCR dietary strategy [35]. This study was beautifully conducted because of the length and employing the BDCR comparison group. The alternate day fasting group was instructed to eat 25% of their daily calories on the fast day, and then eat normally on the feast day. The BDCR group was put on a 25% calorie reduction (see chapter 4) each day for the entirety of the study. ___At the end of the 6 months, both groups lost an average of 7% of their body weight or 14 -16 lbs.___ Similarly, at the end of 12 months ___weight loss was not different between the groups with nearly 12 lbs. lost in both at the end of the study___. This demonstrates that both were effective for weight loss, and that alternate day fasting is safe as a year-long dietary approach.

Now, there were some very important takeaways from this longer duration study. The dropout rate was higher in the alternate day fasting (dropout rate = 38%) group compared to the BDCR group (dropout rate = 28%). Many in the alternate day fasting group cited dissatisfaction with the diet as their reason for withdrawing from the study. This indicates that the strategy may not be suitable to all people who are trying to lose weight, but it does appear to be safe and effective. Alternatively, some people may like the ability to eat unrestricted every other day and use this as motivation to get through the fasting days.

Another important finding in regard to alternate day fasting is that participants appear to not over eat on their "feast" day. In fact, people tended to eat less during their "feast" day. Overeating seems like a natural response that may occur because of the large reduction in food intake during the previous day. In the morning after a fasting day, one may be extremely hungry and consume a large breakfast. The high satiety, or fullness from the large breakfast may lead to lower food intake during the rest of day. This conclusion is purely speculation as food consumption patterns are unknown among people undergoing alternate day fasting diets.

Similar to both the BDCR and meal timing dietary strategies, people who have undergone weight loss through alternate day fasting also demonstrated improvements in markers of metabolism. These included lower levels of circulating triglycerides, glucose, insulin, and A1c [35].

I would like to briefly mention another fasting dietary approach that has been briefly studied and consists of combining intermittent fasting with BDCR. In this strategy, a one day per week fast is added into the BDCR dietary strategy in the effort to accelerate weight loss [42]. Using this combination approach, obese research participants lost between 5 to 10 lbs. in a 7-week time frame. Intermittent fasting has also been added into normal calorie consumption diets to promote weight loss. Here, someone will fast (consuming 400-500 calories) on two consecutive days per week followed by resuming their normal diet for remaining five days per week [43, 44]. Originally, I was going to devote an entire chapter to intermittent fasting in this manual, however I decided against as the approach is very similar to alternative day fasting.

You may have questions about the dietary composition of the food during the fast day. In research studies, fruit juice containing high amounts of carbohydrate has been used, along with a standard recommended breakdown of nutrients containing 30% of energy from fat, 55% from carbohydrate, and 15% from protein [35]. It may be more appropriate to consume a higher percentage of protein and fat during the fasting period to help prevent feelings of hunger. Also, a higher protein intake during the fasting day may help prevent the loss of fat free mass (muscle tissue) during weight loss. It is very important that I state that no research studies have been conducted on high protein intake during fasting diets. Therefore, my comments here are purely speculation, and research studies are needed to evaluate the effectiveness of increasing protein intake during the fast day.

Before we move on, I want to mention that fasting has been practiced among followers of various religions and philosophies. Ramadan is an annual one month fast that is practiced by Muslims to commemorate Islam. Some Christians fast during the 40-day Lent period. In a small study, researchers followed a group of Muslims during Ramadan and observed significant weight lost (up to 8 lbs.) during the monthly fast [45]. Besides this work, little is known about how religious periods of fasting impact the body, but we do know that billions of people worldwide follow the practice, so safety has been established. Because of the relatively new introduction of fasting into the weight loss realm, the safety of long-term fasting remains unknown. This point has been raised by researchers, I only highlight this because I want to be honest with you [46].

Developing the strategy

Adopting and developing the alternate day fasting strategy is rather simple as it doesn't require a great deal of meal planning because you will eat unrestricted on your feast day. Again, I have provided you with an example, and have also provided additional space for you to make calculations.

Example:
Female
34-years old
Lightly active (PA level of 1.12, see Chapter 3, Eq. 3.2)
Body weight: 179 lbs.
Height: 63 inches (5 feet, 3 inches)

Step 1. Metabolic rate = 1,660 calories per day. This was determined based on gender, age, and current weight. Also factored in is the person's daily activity level (PA = 1.12).

Step 2. Calculate fasting day calorie intake.
    25% of energy requirement = 1,660 x .25 = 415 calories.

Step 3. Fasting day calorie intake = 415 calories.

Below is a diet plan for this example.

Table 6.1. Example diet plan for fasting day.

Food description	Nutrient breakdown (estimations)	Calories
Breakfast = 150 calories goal (7am)		
Oatmeal instant maple brown sugar	2g fat, 4g pro, 32g cho	160
Coffee (with cream)	NA	0
	Total	**160**
Lunch = 200 calories goal (12am)		
Protein bar	7g fat, 14g pro, 23g cho	210
Diet soda	NA	0
	Total	**210**
Late afternoon/early dinner = 100 calories		
Protein shake 1 scoop + water	3g fat, 12g pro, 7g cho	100
	Total	**100**
Daily calorie total	**12g fat, 30g pro, 62g cho**	**470**

g-grams, pro-protein, cho-carbohydrate. Total fat calories = 108, total protein calories = 120, and total carbohydrate calories = 248. Calorie totals may not equal nutrient totals due to estimations.

The dietary example in table 6.1 provides 25% of the daily calories from protein during the fasting day, which is considered a higher protein diet. However, the overall amount of protein ingested (30 g.) for this person is far below the recommended intake of 0.8 grams per kilogram body weight, or 65 grams. This is expected simply because of the severe calorie restriction during the fasting day. I must mention that if you're feeling extremely hungry then increase your fasting day calorie intake. I have not provided a dietary log example for the feast day because food intake is as desired.

Alternate day fasting strategy for person with a TEE = 1,660 calories

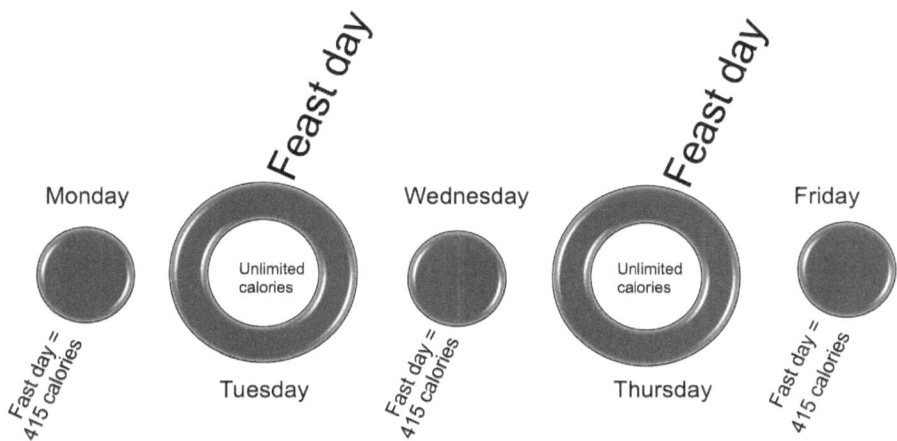

Figure 6.1. Alternate day fasting. This person has a metabolic rate of 1,660 and will consume 25% of their energy needs during each fasting day (Monday, Wednesday, Friday). Feast days will occur on Tuesday and Thursdays. Keep in mind that each week will fluctuate, meaning that fasting days will occur on Tuesday and Thursday during the next week, and feast days will be on Monday, Wednesday, and Friday.

Use the steps below to calculate your own alternate day fasting strategy. I have greyed out the areas for you to complete the calculations.

Step 1. Calculate metabolic rate.

Age: _____.

Height: _____ in.

Body weight: _____ lbs.

Perform the calculation using the equations below and your PA from table 6.2.

Men	TEE or metabolic rate = PA x [(4.5454 x weight in lbs.) + (15.875 x height inches) – (5 x age) +5]
Women	TEE or metabolic rate = PA x [(4.5454 x weight in lbs.) + (15.875 x height inches) – (5 x age) – 161]

Table 6.2. Physical activity (PA) factor

Level	Male	Female
Sedentary – no daily exercise, desk job	1.0	1.0
Light – walking, some physical nature to occupation	1.13	1.12
Moderate – exercise 3-4 times per week for 30-60 minutes. Physical occupation	1.25	1.27
Very active – heavy exercise 7 times per week. Highly physical job (wildland firefighting, heavy construction)	1.48	1.45

Your calculated TEE or metabolic rate = [   ] calories per day.

Remember, this is your calculated metabolic rate

Step 2. Calculate fasting day calorie intake.

25% of energy requirement = TEE or metabolic rate (step 1) x .25% = [   ] daily calorie intake.

Step 3. Fasting day calorie intake = [   ] calories.

Step 4. Develop a tentative meal plan for fasting day.

Nutrition calculators are available online to assist you designing your diet. It is challenging to create and follow a daily food diet. I suggest creating an example of the types and amounts of food you will be able to eat during the fasting day. This will inform you about various foods that you may want to include. Additional blank food logs are available in appendix F.

Table 6.3. Blank food log for fasting day.

Food description	Nutrient breakdown (estimations)	Calories
Breakfast = _____ calories goal		
	Total =	
Lunch = _____ calories goal		
	Total =	
Dinner = _____ calories goal		
	Total =	
Daily totals =		

Step 5. Readjust diet based on weight loss.

I suggest repeating steps 1-4 every 6-weeks. As you lose weight, your metabolic rate will decrease, so to maintain weight loss you will need to adjust your fasting day calorie intake.

Pros and cons

As you may see, the alternate day fasting strategy is much easier to implement than the BDCR and meal timing approaches. While fasting has been practiced for centuries in various religions, the use as a weight loss method is rather new. Therefore, the safety of long term alternate day fasting is not known. However, this approach may present a motivational aspect in that you are faced with the challenge of the fasting day while using the following day (feast day) as motivation to stay committed to the fast. Table 7.4 details several pros and cons to the alternate day fasting strategy.

Table 6.4. Pros and cons of alternate day fasting dietary strategy

Pros	Cons
Effective for weight loss in short-term studies (12 to 26 weeks).	Longer duration (> 1 year) studies do not exist, so long-term safety and sustainability are unknown.
Weight loss ranges between 6 to 16 lbs.	Some research participants have stated their dissatisfaction during the fasting days.
The ability to eat unrestricted may provide motivation to get through the fasting days.	May be difficult to maintain as dropout rates have been reported at 38%.
Easier to maintain dietary log during fasting day.	Inadequate nutrient intake during fasting days.
May be easily combined with other weight loss strategies such as BDCR.	Participants may be prone to over eating during feast day.
Body fat and body mass index decrease.	
Improvement in markers of metabolism (e.g., blood glucose, insulin, A1c).	

Chapter 7. The role of exercise

Exercise becomes especially important in a weight loss program. One reason is to offset the calorie restriction goal. Let me explain. In a 25% calorie reduction study, a sub group of participants were asked to cut 12.5% by adjusting their diet, and to increase calorie expenditure by 12.5% though exercise to reach the 25% reduction goal [28]. This group lost the same amount of weight (nearly 10% body weight) at 6 months as the group that cut 25% through diet alone. If your 25% goal is a reduction of 500 calories per day then you would simply reduce energy intake by 250 calories and burn 250 calories through exercise each day.

You may be asking how much exercise this would require? If a 250 lb. person walks on a treadmill at 3 mph and 2% grade for 30 minutes they will burn roughly 250 calories. If this same person cycles on a stationary bike for 30 minutes at 88 watts they will burn 262 calories. As you may notice, this is not an unattainable amount of exercise. In fact, if you already participate in weekly sporting activity, such as softball, tennis, golf, basketball, or soccer then you're most likely reaching your calorie expenditure goals. If you're unable to exercise every day then a solid schedule is to use the split approach (diet combined with exercise) during 3-4 days per week and use the diet alone approach for the remaining days.

Several recent news articles and research publications have indicated that exercise alone is not a great weight loss strategy [47]. I agree with these findings because you can exercise for 30-60 minutes and expend between 250-500 calories and quickly abolish this by eating five cookies. In fact, it has been recommended that one needs to exercise between 60-90 minutes per day for it to be effective as a sole weight loss strategy [47]. Very few people have the both the time and motivation to commit to this type of exercise regimen. However, as mentioned previously, it is ideal to add exercise into any of the weight loss strategies mentioned in this manual, and the exercise does not need to be rigorous or unenjoyable. A 30-60-minute daily walk or bike ride, or a participation in a group exercise class are all easily implemented into daily life. Please keep in mind that the benefits of exercise extend far beyond it as a component in a weight loss strategy. Consistent exercise promotes heart, metabolic, skeletal muscle, and psychological health; and ultimately delays the aging process. In fact, exercise is considered the number one disease prevention activity that one can par-take in on a daily basis [48, 49].

Another extremely important reason to include exercise into your diet is to preserve muscle mass. A common occurrence during weight loss is a decrease in muscle tissue. When you're in a calorie deficit each day, your body will breakdown tissue to provide nutrients to the body, and both fat and muscle will be broken down. To prevent this from occurring, I highly suggest participating in resistance (weight training) exercise. In studies where participants are asked to perform weight training exercise 2-3 times per week while in a calorie deficit, they routinely preserve muscle mass, and ultimately lose more fat mass. This can be accomplished by performing 30-40 minutes of resistance exercise 2-3 times per week. Using machine weights, or body weight exercises is perfectly suitable; or, you may want to enroll in exercise classes such as cross training. You do not have to be a hardcore weight lifter. Here is an example of a simple, but effective weight training program.

Table 7.1. Resistance training example.

Weight training exercise	Number of sets	Repetitions	Effort level
Leg press	2-3	10-15	Challenging
Leg extension	2-3	10-15	Challenging
Chest press	2-3	10-15	Challenging
Lat pulldowns	2-3	10-15	Challenging
Leg curl	2-3	10-15	Challenging
Shoulder press	2-3	10-15	Challenging
Abdominal exercise	2-3	20-30	Challenging

Sets = the number of times you perform the exercise; Repetitions = the number of times you lift the weight during each set; Effort level = how hard the exercise feels to you.

When overweight men and women participated in resistance exer-cise during a very low-calorie diet that included only 800 calories per day, they lost fat weight and preserved muscle tissue. In fact, they even increased muscle tissue, which was a big surprise to the research team [50].

A blossoming area of study in the field of physical activity is called non-exercise activity thermogenesis, or NEAT, which is the amount of activity you perform during the day that is not specifically planned ex-ercise. Simply stated, this is the amount of time you spend doing anything but sitting, and includes simple movements such as standing, walking, cleaning, or yard work. You see, sitting is the root of all evil (kidding) because it is a state where a small number of calories are being burned. Unfortunately, we spend an enormous percentage of our day in a seated or lying position. In fact, every additional hour per day of TV watching (commonly performed in a sitting or lying position) has been associated with an increased risk of mortality from chronic inflammatory disease such as heart disease [51]. What has been revealed in regards to NEAT is that you can burn nearly 350 calories per day by increasing your time standing, walking, and even fidgeting [52]. Many people have embraced activity tracking devices (e.g., Fitbits, fitness watches) that estimate calories burned each day based on movement. Researchers have highlighted health benefits such as decreased body mass index and blood pressure by achieving 10,000 steps per day [53]. In fact, it has been recently reported that those people who engage in nearly 10,000 steps per day are more likely to successfully lose 10% body weight (20 lbs. for a 200 lb. person) during a 6-month diet, and sustain the weight loss at 18 months [54]. I believe this highlights the added benefit of daily low intensity physical activity on weight loss and management.

A brilliant expert in the field of exercise physiology, and a close mentor of mine, frequently lectures on the topic of NEAT. He routinely will ask his audience to write down on a piece paper how many hours per day they spend sitting, and will discuss simple ways to decrease inactivity, or sitting time [55]. Suggestions include:

- Standing whenever possible (at work, in meetings, on the train, at home).
- Walking your dog.
- Walking around your neighborhood or at a local park.
- Wash your car by hand.
- Pace sideline at your child's sporting event.
- Walk all of the aisles when grocery shopping.
- Park at the furthest parking spot from your office.
- Get up and walk after 30 minutes of sitting.
- When shopping, walk around stores or malls.
- Take a 30-minute lunch and spend remaining 30 minutes walking.
- Pace the airport while waiting for your flight.

Below I have highlighted general aerobic exercise recommendations as stated by the American College of Sports Medicine (ACSM). General exercise recommendations include [56].

- Frequency: 3-5 days per week.
- Intensity: Moderate to vigorous, which ranges between 6 (moderate) to 8 (vigorous) on a 0-10-point scale.
- Duration per session: accumulate at least 30 minutes and up to 60 minutes per exercise session, or a total of 150-300 minutes per week.
- Type: any mode of exercise that you enjoy such as walking, cycling, group fitness, or aquatic exercise.

Unfortunately, the majority of people regardless of nationality do not meet these goals each week. These recommendations are focused on aerobic activities; however, other types of exercise modalities exist, and are encouraged. Many of these activities incorporate both cardiovascular and muscle strengthening exercises. I have provided several examples below, but the list could be nearly endless.

- Resistance exercise (see above).
- Yoga exercise.
- Circuit training exercise.
- Martial arts classes.
- Rock climbing.

The biggest challenge that we have in the field of exercise physiology is motivating people to exercise. We can conduct endless research studies demonstrating the multitude of benefits from engaging in a consistent exercise regimen, but we have yet to develop a system or intervention among humans that leads to sustained participation in exercise. I liken exercise to brushing your teeth in that it is a daily habit because you do not want your teeth to rot. Exercise or physical movement should be a daily activity to prevent your body from rotting (I know it is a little extreme). Keep in mind that exercise should be enjoyable. Daily walking is adequate enough to meet the exercise recommendations previously stated above. I enjoy walking and commonly walk on a treadmill for 45-60 minutes while I watch a show on

Netflix. I find it to be an enjoyable break from the business of life, and I feel refreshed afterwards.

Remember, exercise is a fantastic supplement into any of previously discussed weight loss strategies. Burning an extra 250-500 calories per day will create a larger daily calorie deficit leading to heightened weight loss. In addition, by reducing the amount of time sitting will also increase daily energy expenditure and will further widen your daily calorie deficit.

Conclusions

My goal for this manual is to bring evidence-based weight loss strategies into daily practice. Millions of dollars are spent throughout the world to fund weight loss research. Unfortunately, much of the positive outcomes get buried in scientific journals that have limited readership. To conduct human subject studies, researchers must follow strict guidelines, and therefore results are grounded in safety and statistics. Simply stated, research must protect participants (safe dietary intervention strategies), and results (either positive or negative) must have statistical support. In the previous chapters in this manual I have attempted to inform and guide you in developing weight loss strategies that are grounded in science.

In the appendices that follow, I have provided blank documents to assist in calculating your metabolic rate and developing your dietary log for each strategy. I have also included helpful websites for nutrient tracking and diet recommendations.

Before I sign off, I would thank you for taking time to read this manual. I hope that you have found the content interesting and most importantly, valuable. I will continually update this manual as new evidence-based weight loss strategies are developed and tested. However, I am confident that if you are able to incorporate one the strategies previously discussed and combine it with daily physical activity then you will lose weight. It will take effort and there will be times when you over indulge when celebrating a life event or in social arenas. It is ok, don't beat yourself up. Weight loss occurs over time, so if you're able to consistently sustain a calorie deficit then weight loss will occur.

Best of luck, and please keep me posted on your success.

Appendices

Appendix A. Simple dietary approaches to reduce calorie intake.

Appendix B. Helpful websites for nutrient tracking and diet advice.

Appendix C. Calculating your metabolic rate.

Appendix D. Balanced daily calorie restriction (BDCR) diet strategy blank food logs.

Appendix E. Meal timing diet blank food logs.

Appendix F. Alternate day fasting diet strategy blank food logs.

Appendix A. Simple dietary approaches to reduce calorie intake

Below I have listed several dietary decisions that you can make to reduce daily calorie intake:

- Do not drink your calories. Try to drink water, or non-calorie drinks.
- When feeling hungry, drink a glass of water, or some other non-calorie drink (e.g., diet soda, flavored carbonated water, or coffee/tea.
- Try to consume low energy dense foods such as vegetables, fruits, and other high fiber foods.
- Higher protein meals may increase your sense of fullness and decrease hunger.
- Drink more water.
- Try to cook with lower calorie oils or sprays.
- Try to reduce eating out.
- Reduce alcohol consumption.
- Get adequate sleep.
- Smaller portions.

Appendix B. Helpful websites for nutrient tracking and diet advice

Below are several websites or apps that may assist you with nutrient tracking:

www.myfitnesspal.com.
www.fatsecret.com.

Below are several websites that provide weight loss tips and healthy advice:

www.nutrition.gov.
www.cdc.gov/healthyweight.
www.heart.org/HEARTORG/healthyliving.
www.eatright.org.

Appendix C. Calculating your metabolic rate

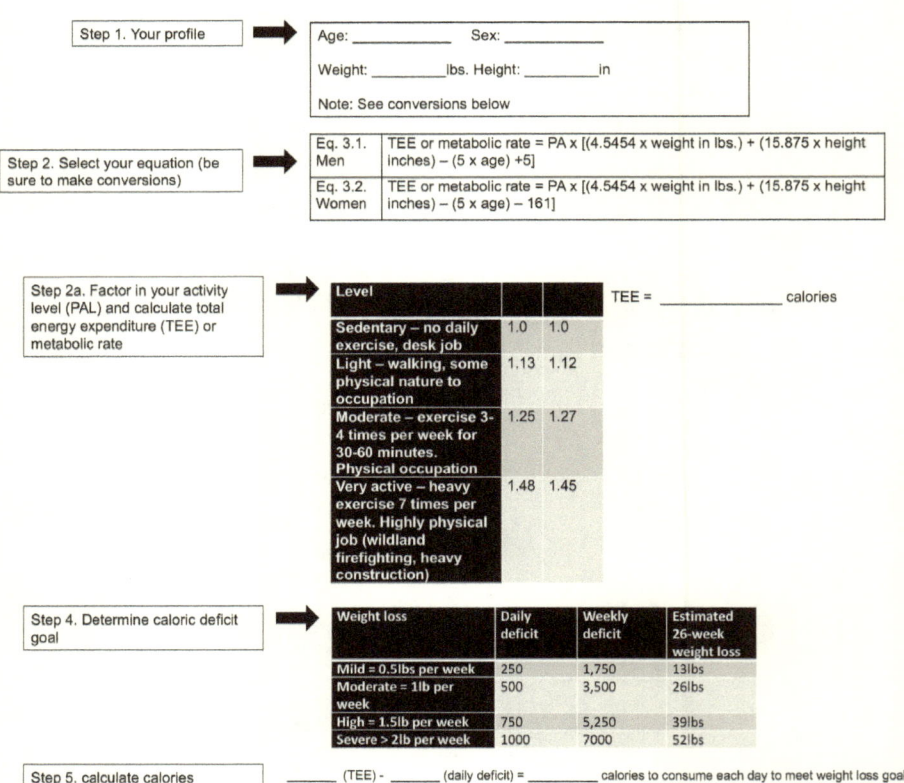

Step 1. Your profile

Age: _____ Sex: _____

Weight: _____lbs. Height: _____in

Note: See conversions below

Step 2. Select your equation (be sure to make conversions)

| Eq. 3.1. Men | TEE or metabolic rate = PA x [(4.5454 x weight in lbs.) + (15.875 x height inches) – (5 x age) +5] |
| Eq. 3.2. Women | TEE or metabolic rate = PA x [(4.5454 x weight in lbs.) + (15.875 x height inches) – (5 x age) – 161] |

Step 2a. Factor in your activity level (PAL) and calculate total energy expenditure (TEE) or metabolic rate

TEE = _____ calories

Level		
Sedentary – no daily exercise, desk job	1.0	1.0
Light – walking, some physical nature to occupation	1.13	1.12
Moderate – exercise 3-4 times per week for 30-60 minutes. Physical occupation	1.25	1.27
Very active – heavy exercise 7 times per week. Highly physical job (wildland firefighting, heavy construction)	1.48	1.45

Step 4. Determine caloric deficit goal

Weight loss	Daily deficit	Weekly deficit	Estimated 26-week weight loss
Mild = 0.5lbs per week	250	1,750	13lbs
Moderate = 1lb per week	500	3,500	26lbs
High = 1.5lb per week	750	5,250	39lbs
Severe > 2lb per week	1000	7000	52lbs

Step 5. calculate calories

_____ (TEE) - _____ (daily deficit) = _____ calories to consume each day to meet weight loss goal

Appendix D. Balanced daily calorie restriction (BDCR) diet strategy blank food logs

Food description	Nutrient breakdown (estimations)	Calories
Meal 1 = _____ calories goal (7am)		
	Total	=
Meal 2 = _____ calories goal (11am)		
	Total	=
Meal 3 = _____ calories goal (3pm)		
	Total	=
Meal 4 = _____ calories goal (7pm)		
	Total	=
Daily total		=

Food description	Nutrient breakdown (estimations)	Calories
Meal 1 = _____ calories goal (7am)		
	Total	=
Meal 2 = _____ calories goal (11am)		
	Total	=
Meal 3 = _____ calories goal (3pm)		
	Total	=
Meal 4 = _____ calories goal (7pm)		
	Total	=
Daily total		=

Appendix E. Meal timing diet blank food logs

High breakfast meal timing strategy:

    Breakfast, 51% of calories = _____ calories

    Lunch, 35% of calories = _____calories

    Dinner, 14% of calories = _____calories

High dinner meal timing strategy

    Breakfast, 14% of calories = _____calories

    Lunch, 35% of calories = _____calories

    Dinner, 51% of calories = _____calories

Table 5.3. Blank food log for meal timing strategy

Food description	Nutrient breakdown (estimations)	Calories
Breakfast = _____ calories goal		
	Total	
Lunch = _____ calories goal		
	Total	
Dinner = _____ calories goal		
	Total	
Daily totals		

Food description	Nutrient breakdown (estimations)	Calories
Breakfast =_____ calories goal		
	Total	
Lunch =_____ calories goal		
	Total	
Dinner =_____ calories goal		
	Total	
Daily totals		

Appendix F. Alternate day fasting diet strategy blank food logs

The goal is to take in roughly 25% of TEE needs during the fasting days (see figure 3.1 to estimate TEE).

25% of energy requirement = TEE or metabolic rate x .25% = _____ daily calorie intake.

Food description	Nutrient breakdown (estimations)	Calories
Breakfast = _____ calories goal		
	Total =	
Lunch = _____ calories goal		
	Total =	
Dinner = _____ calories goal		
	Total =	
Daily totals =		

Food description	Nutrient breakdown (estimations)	Calories
Breakfast = _____ calories goal		
	Total =	
Lunch = _____ calories goal		
	Total =	
Dinner = _____ calories goal		
	Total =	
Daily totals =		

References

1. Weiss, E.C., D.A. Galuska, L.K. Khan, and M.K. Serdula, Weight-control practices among US adults, 2001–2002. *American journal of preventive medicine*, 2006. 31(1): p. 18-24.

2. Serdula, M.K., A.H. Mokdad, D.F. Williamson, D.A. Galuska, J.M. Mendlein, and G.W. Heath, Prevalence of attempting weight loss and strategies for controlling weight. *Jama*, 1999. 282(14): p. 1353-1358.

3. Gardner, C.D., A. Kiazand, S. Alhassan, S. Kim, R.S. Stafford, R.R. Balise, et al., Comparison of the Atkins, Zone, Ornish, and LEARN diets for change in weight and related risk factors among overweight premenopausal women: the A TO Z Weight Loss Study: a randomized trial. *Jama*, 2007. 297(9): p. 969-977.

4. Soenen, S., A.G. Bonomi, S.G. Lemmens, J. Scholte, M.A. Thijssen, F. van Berkum, et al., Relatively high-protein or 'low-carb'energy-restricted diets for body weight loss and body weight maintenance? *Physiology & behavior*, 2012. 107(3): p. 374-380.

5. Sacks, F.M., G.A. Bray, V.J. Carey, S.R. Smith, D.H. Ryan, S.D. Anton, et al., Comparison of weight-loss diets with different compositions of fat, protein, and carbohydrates. *New England Journal of Medicine*, 2009. 360(9): p. 859-873.

6. Björntorp, P. and L. Sjöström, Number and size of adipose tissue fat cells in relation to metabolism in human obesity. *Metabolism-Clinical and Experimental*, 1971. 20(7): p. 703-713.

7. Meerman, R. and A.J. Brown, When somebody loses weight, where does the fat go? *Bmj*, 2014. 349: p. g7257.

8. Finkler, E., S.B. Heymsfield, and M.-P. St-Onge, Rate of weight loss can be predicted by patient characteristics and intervention strategies. *Journal of the Academy of Nutrition and Dietetics*, 2012. 112(1): p. 75-80.

9. National Heart, L. and B. Institute, Clinical guidelines on the identification, evaluation, and treatment of overweight and obesity in adults (NIH Publication No. 98-4083). *National Institutes of Health*, 1998.

10. Mifflin, M.D., S.T. St Jeor, L.A. Hill, B.J. Scott, S.A. Daugherty, and Y.O. Koh, A new predictive equation for resting energy expenditure in healthy individuals. *The American journal of clinical nutrition*, 1990. 51(2): p. 241-247.

11. Tang, M., C.L. Armstrong, H.J. Leidy, and W.W. Campbell, Normal vs. high-protein weight loss diets in men: Effects on body composition and indices of metabolic syndrome. *Obesity*, 2013. 21(3): p. E204-E210.

12. Mutch, D.M., M.R. Temanni, C. Henegar, F. Combes, V. Pelloux, C. Holst, et al., Adipose gene expression prior to weight loss can differentiate and weakly predict dietary responders. *PloS one*, 2007. 2(12): p. e1344.

13. Atkins, R.C., *Dr. Atkins' diet revolution*. 1981: Bantam Books New York.

14. Health, U.D.o. and H. Services, *Dietary guidelines for Americans 2015-2020*. 2017: Skyhorse Publishing Inc.

15. Eisenstein, J., S.B. Roberts, G. Dallal, and E. Saltzman, High-protein weight-loss diets: are they safe and do they work? A review of the experimental and epidemiologic data. *Nutrition reviews*, 2002. 60(7): p. 189-200.

16. Clifton, P.M., J.B. Keogh, and M. Noakes, Long-term effects of a high-protein weight-loss diet–. *The American journal of clinical nutrition*, 2008. 87(1): p. 23-29.

17. Skov, A., S. Toubro, B. Rønn, L. Holm, and A. Astrup, Randomized trial on protein vs carbohydrate in ad libitum fat reduced diet for the treatment of obesity. *International journal of obesity*, 1999. 23(5): p. 528.

18. Halton, T.L. and F.B. Hu, The effects of high protein diets on thermogenesis, satiety and weight loss: a critical review. *Journal of the American College of Nutrition*, 2004. 23(5): p. 373-385.

19. Campos-Nonato, I., L. Hernandez, and S. Barquera, Effect of a high-protein diet versus standard-protein diet on weight loss and biomarkers of metabolic syndrome: a randomized clinical trial. *Obesity facts*, 2017. 10(3): p. 238-251.

20. Krieger, J.W., H.S. Sitren, M.J. Daniels, and B. Langkamp-Henken, Effects of variation in protein and carbohydrate intake on body mass and composition during energy restriction: a meta-

regression–. *The American journal of clinical nutrition*, 2006. 83(2): p. 260-274.

21. Paoli, A., A. Rubini, J. Volek, and K. Grimaldi, Beyond weight loss: a review of the therapeutic uses of very-low-carbohydrate (ketogenic) diets. *European journal of clinical nutrition*, 2013. 67(8): p. 789.

22. Astrup, A., T.M. Larsen, and A. Harper, Atkins and other low-carbohydrate diets: hoax or an effective tool for weight loss? *The Lancet*, 2004. 364(9437): p. 897-899.

23. Westerterp-Plantenga, M., A. Nieuwenhuizen, D. Tome, S. Soenen, and K. Westerterp, Dietary protein, weight loss, and weight maintenance. *Annual review of nutrition*, 2009. 29: p. 21-41.

24. Westman, E.C., R.D. Feinman, J.C. Mavropoulos, M.C. Vernon, J.S. Volek, J.A. Wortman, et al., Low-carbohydrate nutrition and metabolism–. *The American journal of clinical nutrition*, 2007. 86(2): p. 276-284.

25. Ebbeling, C.B., J.F. Swain, H.A. Feldman, W.W. Wong, D.L. Hachey, E. Garcia-Lago, et al., Effects of dietary composition on energy expenditure during weight-loss maintenance. *Jama*, 2012. 307(24): p. 2627-2634.

26. Jon Schoenfeld, B., A. Albert Aragon, and J.W. Krieger, Effects of meal frequency on weight loss and body composition: a meta-analysis. *Nutrition reviews*, 2015. 73(2): p. 69-82.

27. Kulovitz, M.G., L.R. Kravitz, C. Mermier, A.L. Gibson, C.A. Conn, D. Kolkmeyer, et al., Potential role of meal frequency as a strategy for weight loss and health in overweight or obese adults. *Nutrition*, 2014. 30(4): p. 386-392.

28. Heilbronn, L.K., L. de Jonge, M.I. Frisard, J.P. DeLany, D.E. Larson-Meyer, J. Rood, et al., Effect of 6-month calorie restriction on biomarkers of longevity, metabolic adaptation, and oxidative stress in overweight individuals: a randomized controlled trial. *Jama*, 2006. 295(13): p. 1539-1548.

29. Lichtenstein, A.H., L.J. Appel, M. Brands, M. Carnethon, S. Daniels, H.A. Franch, et al., Diet and lifestyle recommendations revision 2006: a scientific statement from the American Heart Association Nutrition Committee. *Circulation*, 2006. 114(1): p. 82-96.

30. Brehm, B.J., R.J. Seeley, S.R. Daniels, and D.A. D'alessio, A randomized trial comparing a very low carbohydrate diet and a calorie-restricted low fat diet on body weight and cardiovascular risk factors in healthy women. *The Journal of Clinical Endocrinology & Metabolism*, 2003. 88(4): p. 1617-1623.

31. Wadden, T.A., G.D. Foster, and K.A. Letizia, One-year behavioral treatment of obesity: comparison of moderate and severe caloric restriction and the effects of weight maintenance therapy. *Journal of consulting and clinical psychology*, 1994. 62(1): p. 165.

32. Saris, W.H., Very-low-calorie diets and sustained weight loss. *Obesity research*, 2001. 9(S11): p. 295S-301S.

33. Wing, R.R., E.H. Blair, P. Bononi, M.D. Marcus, R. Watanabe, and R.N. Bergman, Caloric restriction per se is a significant factor in improvements in glycemic control and insulin sensitivity during weight loss in obese NIDDM patients. *Diabetes care*, 1994. 17(1): p. 30-36.

34. Larson-Meyer, D.E., L.K. Heilbronn, L.M. Redman, B.R. Newcomer, M.I. Frisard, S. Anton, et al., Effect of calorie restriction with or without exercise on insulin sensitivity, β-cell function, fat cell size, and ectopic lipid in overweight subjects. *Diabetes care*, 2006. 29(6): p. 1337-1344.

35. Trepanowski, J.F., C.M. Kroeger, A. Barnosky, M.C. Klempel, S. Bhutani, K.K. Hoddy, et al., Effect of alternate-day fasting on weight loss, weight maintenance, and cardioprotection among metabolically healthy obese adults: a randomized clinical trial. *JAMA internal medicine*, 2017. 177(7): p. 930-938.

36. Jakubowicz, D., M. Barnea, J. Wainstein, and O. Froy, High caloric intake at breakfast vs. dinner differentially influences weight loss of overweight and obese women. *Obesity*, 2013. 21(12): p. 2504-2512.

37. Rabinovitz, H.R., M. Boaz, T. Ganz, D. Jakubowicz, Z. Matas, Z. Madar, et al., Big breakfast rich in protein and fat improves glycemic control in type 2 diabetics. *Obesity*, 2014. 22(5): p. E46-E54.

38. Garaulet, M., P. Gómez-Abellán, J.J. Alburquerque-Béjar, Y.-C. Lee, J.M. Ordovás, and F.A. Scheer, Timing of food intake

predicts weight loss effectiveness. *International journal of obesity*, 2013. 37(4): p. 604.

39. Weigle, D.S., P.A. Breen, C.C. Matthys, H.S. Callahan, K.E. Meeuws, V.R. Burden, et al., A high-protein diet induces sustained reductions in appetite, ad libitum caloric intake, and body weight despite compensatory changes in diurnal plasma leptin and ghrelin concentrations–. *The American journal of clinical nutrition*, 2005. 82(1): p. 41-48.

40. Varady, K.A., S. Bhutani, M.C. Klempel, C.M. Kroeger, J.F. Trepanowski, J.M. Haus, et al., Alternate day fasting for weight loss in normal weight and overweight subjects: a randomized controlled trial. *Nutrition journal*, 2013. 12(1): p. 146.

41. Hoddy, K.K., C.M. Kroeger, J.F. Trepanowski, A. Barnosky, S. Bhutani, and K.A. Varady, Meal timing during alternate day fasting: Impact on body weight and cardiovascular disease risk in obese adults. *Obesity*, 2014. 22(12): p. 2524-2531.

42. Klempel, M.C., C.M. Kroeger, S. Bhutani, J.F. Trepanowski, and K.A. Varady, Intermittent fasting combined with calorie restriction is effective for weight loss and cardio-protection in obese women. *Nutrition journal*, 2012. 11(1): p. 98.

43. Barnosky, A.R., K.K. Hoddy, T.G. Unterman, and K.A. Varady, Intermittent fasting vs daily calorie restriction for type 2 diabetes prevention: a review of human findings. *Translational Research*, 2014. 164(4): p. 302-311.

44. Tinsley, G.M. and P.M. La Bounty, Effects of intermittent fasting on body composition and clinical health markers in humans. *Nutrition reviews*, 2015. 73(10): p. 661-674.

45. Ziaee, V., M. Razaei, Z. Ahmadinejad, H. Shaikh, R. Yousefi, L. Yarmohammadi, et al., The changes of metabolic profile and weight during Ramadan fasting. *Singapore medical journal*, 2006. 47(5): p. 409.

46. Horne, B.D., J.B. Muhlestein, and J.L. Anderson, Health effects of intermittent fasting: hormesis or harm? A systematic review. *The American journal of clinical nutrition*, 2015. 102(2): p. 464-470.

47. Swift, D.L., N.M. Johannsen, C.J. Lavie, C.P. Earnest, and T.S. Church, The role of exercise and physical activity in weight loss and maintenance. *Progress in cardiovascular diseases*, 2014. 56(4): p. 441-447.

48. Nelson, M.E., W.J. Rejeski, S.N. Blair, P.W. Duncan, J.O. Judge, A.C. King, et al., Physical activity and public health in older adults: recommendation from the American College of Sports Medicine and the American Heart Association. *Circulation*, 2007. 116(9): p. 1094.

49. Kohl 3rd, H.W., C.L. Craig, E.V. Lambert, S. Inoue, J.R. Alkandari, G. Leetongin, et al., The pandemic of physical inactivity: global action for public health. *The Lancet*, 2012. 380(9838): p. 294-305.

50. Verreijen, A.M., S. Verlaan, M.F. Engberink, S. Swinkels, J. de Vogel-van den Bosch, and P.J. Weijs, A high whey protein–, leucine-, and vitamin D–enriched supplement preserves muscle mass during intentional weight loss in obese older adults: a double-blind randomized controlled trial–. *The American journal of clinical nutrition*, 2014. 101(2): p. 279-286.

51. Grace, M.S., F. Dillon, E.L. Barr, S.K. Keadle, N. Owen, and D.W. Dunstan, Television Viewing Time and Inflammatory-Related Mortality. *Medicine and science in sports and exercise*, 2017. 49(10): p. 2040-2047.

52. von Loeffelholz, C., The role of non-exercise activity thermogenesis in human obesity. 2014.

53. Schneider, P.L., D.R. Bassett Jr, D.L. Thompson, N.P. Pronk, and K.M. Bielak, Effects of a 10,000 steps per day goal in overweight adults. *American Journal of Health Promotion*, 2006. 21(2): p. 85-89.

54. Creasy, S.A., W. Lang, D.F. Tate, K.K. Davis, and J.M. Jakicic, Pattern of Daily Steps is Associated with Weight Loss: Secondary Analysis from the Step-Up Randomized Trial. *Obesity*, 2018. 26(6): p. 977-984.

55. Kravitz, L., A NEAT "new" strategy for weight control. *The Practical Guide to Weight Management, Understanding the Role of Diet, Nutrition, Exercise and Lifestyle*, 2006: p. 14.

56. Medicine, A.C.o.S., *ACSM's guidelines for exercise testing and prescription*. 2013: Lippincott Williams & Wilkins.